This Journal Belongs To

____

www.ingramcontent.com/pod-product-compliance
Lightning Source LLC
Chambersburg PA
CBHW072011280526
45788CB00013B/2313